Healing Through the Ages: A Guide to the Evolution of Wound Care

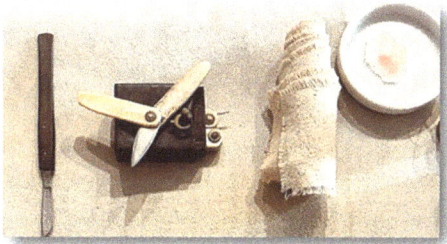

Dr. Christine Miller

Healing Through the Ages: A Guide to the Evolution of Wound Care
by Dr. Christine Miller

This edition published in 2024

Winged Hussar Publishing is an imprint of

Winged Hussar Publishing, LLC
1525 Hulse Rd, Unit 1
Point Pleasant, NJ 08742

Copyright © Winged Hussar Publishing and Dr. Christine Miller
ISBN 978-1-958872-35-2
Bibliographical References and Index
1. History. 2. Medicine. 3. Military

Winged Hussar Publishing, LLC All rights reserved
For more information
visit us at www.whpsupplyroom.com

Twitter: WingHusPubLLC
Facebook: Winged Hussar Publishing LLC

Helpful Glossary

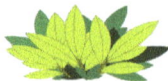

Analgesic	Substance that relieves pain
Antiseptic	Chemical that prevents the growth of disease-causing microorganisms
Astringent	Substance that causes contraction of tissue and dries up secretions
Decoction	Extracting chemicals from hard plant materials (roots & bark)
Diuretic	Substance that increases urination
Emetic	Substance that causes vomiting
Infusion	Extracting oils from delicate parts of the plant (flowers & leaves)
Poultice	A moist mass of plant material wrapped in a cloth
Styptics	Topical substance capable of stopping bleeding

Preface

This book is a highlight of the treatments made over the centuries by medical personnel in the challenging discipline of wound healing and limb preservation. Even with access to advanced technology, and the focus of saving limbs has shifted somewhat as a struggle with diabetes has added another level of complexity in modern society. Please note that many cultures around the world had robust medicinal knowledge! The mention of certain regions and individuals is based off the availability of source documents with respect to all nations and ethnic groups.

This overview at the evolution of healing practices and historically people who influenced them provides a glimpse of innovation but by <u>no means is comprehensive</u>. Contemporary healthcare professionals face different obstacles in the pursuit of healing but can draw inspiration from those who preceded them. Hopefully, the history of healing will appeal to healthcare professionals and history-lovers alike! Modern medicine owes a debt of gratitude to the healers of the past who can be seen as providing building blocks based on the material available to them.

Table of Contents

Healing Through the Ages

Section I: The Ancient Roots of Healing to the Middle Ages

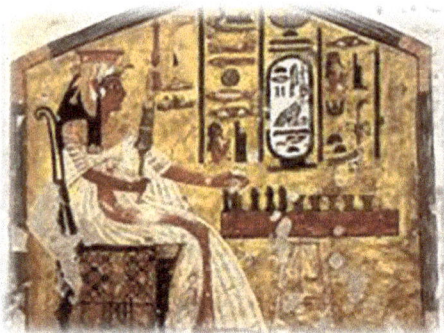

(Image credit: Ancient Egypt, History.com)

There are many ancient cultures who had treatment algorithms or decision trees in place regarding skin ulcerations (wounds), and Egypt in particularly had extensive documentation that has survived to the modern day. The Papyrus of Ebers (Eb) from about 1500 B.C. details the use of warm frog oil directly applied to wounds as a curative measure. The use of frog oil may seem odd to the modern medical knowledge, but these remedies were formed through observations that might rightly or wrongly help healing. In fact, the Egyptians introduced many therapeutically advantageous dressings that are still used in contemporary care. Early on in developing cultures religious belief and healing were strongly linked in ancient traditions.

Egyptian Dressings & Remedies

Understanding the causes of infection (germ theory) would not be fully understood for centuries to come, but the Egyptians had very valuable remedies that did combat infection they developed through observation as well as trial and error. One favorite topical application was honey, and it was mentioned hundreds of times in the Egyptian pharmacopeia. From the modern scientific perspective, honey inhibits the growth of microorganisms which is beneficial to healing in the presence of a wound infection. Animal grease placed on and around the wound bed as a barrier against possible contamination. The use of frankincense, turpentine, and date wine also provided antiseptic properties that aided in the restorative process. A tea made of chamomile (Matricaria chamomilla) has been proven to inhibit the growth of Staphylococcus aureus, a common bacterial cause of skin infections. Matricaria chamomilla tea was a remedy used not only in ancient Egypt but also in Greece, Rome, and India.

A decoction (a method of extracting a liquid through heating or boiling) of willow bark was used in the treatment for a painfully inflamed skin ulceration, the bark itself contains salicin (the active ingredient in Aspirin). The protocol for treating fresh lacerations was to bind the skin edges with adhesive linen strips or sew together with stitches. Wounds were wrapped with linen of varying quality as seen in the mummified bodies exhumed from the ancient tombs. Green copper obtained from malachite applied to wounds provided antiseptic and astringent coverage which enhanced healing and also served as an eye shadow for cosmetic purposes. Mercury and arsenic were incorporated into the Egyptian formulary wound treatment for their antimicrobial properties despite the potential for toxicity. Lemon slices were used to treat burn wounds which would decrease the risk of infection. Imhotep was a famous Egyptian physician (circa 2780 B.C.) who was the medical advisor to pharaoh, Zoster the first king of the Third Dynasty.

Ancient Origins of Biosurgery (Larval Therapy)

The use of insects within the wound bed is expected when there is dead tissue or necrosis, while this is a bit gruesome to the modern sensibility, there are therapeutic benefits to this situation. Maggots produce enzymes that breakdown dead matter without damaging healthy tissue. The larval presence helps accelerate healing by promoting granulation (the formation of connective tissue). The use of maggots in helping to heal wounds is even recorded during biblical times, particularly in the Book of Job (Old Testament). Today, the use of maggots or biosurgery is a practical option in the clinical setting for removing necrotic debris along with the antimicrobial advantages of the larval enzymes.

Ancient Greece & Rome

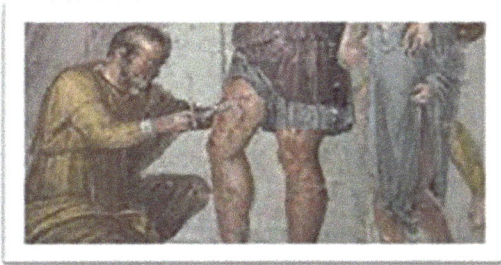

(Image Credit: Worldhistory.org)

The Ancient Greeks & Romans, much like their Egyptian counterparts, perceived medicine as an adjunctive aspect to the true universal healer-nature. Hippocrates, largely regarded as the father of medicine in the Greek and Roman world, viewed the art of healing as individualized to meet the needs of each patient. He wrote several works dating back to the 4th century B.C. (which might have been based on earlier works), and his treatise on Wounds, suggested the presence of pus was a normal part of the healing cascade. This view on pus or suppuration was tied to the idea of "humors" which would stay relevant until the 19th century, ending only after the acceptance of germ theory. Hippocrates did advocate for the use of wine as a wound cleanser which did offer antimicrobial benefits. Turpentine and honey with their antiseptic qualities were also a standard treatment in Greek medicine. Metallic silver was a staple in the ancient world for preserving water and food. Hippocrates applied silver preparations to promote healing in skin ulcerations. Silver continues to be a key antimicrobial agent for the treatment of chronic wounds. Hippocrates would inspire future generations of physicians for centuries to come.

Aulus Cornelius Celsus, Roman encyclopedist, further expanded upon Hippocrates' philosophy regarding the treatment of wounds in the 1st century A.D. Celsus highlighted the importance of controlling bleeding and encouraged the primary closure of fresh wounds with either *sutures* (stitches) or compressive bandaging. He noted that severely burned skin needed to have the dead tissue removed (debridement) for healing to occur. This principle of removing devitalized flesh has carried on through the ages into the modern era. Celsus performed surgical excision of contracted scars for burn wounds. Pedanios Dioscorides, Greek physician, who served in the Roman army recommended honey be applied topically to rotten and hollow ulcers with frequent dressing changes in his extensive work, the *Material Medica*. He also advocated for the use of cow droppings and rose oil for treating burns.

During this period, the disease which caused excessive urination and led to ulcerations of the legs and feet was termed "Diabetes" by Greco-Roman physician, Aretaeus of Cappadocia around the 2nd century A.D. The name Diabetes is derived from the Greek word (diabaino) meaning to "to run through" as a reference to the increased urinary output of patients afflicted with this disorder. Diabetes remains one the main causes of delayed wound healing and subsequent lower extremity amputations in the 21st century.

Claudius Galen, a Greek physician, in the 1st century A.D had a profound and lasting impact on medicine. He built upon the theories of Hippocrates including the concept of the four humors: blood, yellow bile, black bile, and phlegm. The balance of these four humors was the essence wellness and illness were a sign of imbalance. Bloodletting was the go-to 1st line treatment to regain humoral balance. The use of lancets and leeches were common methods of bloodletting, and inducing vomiting was another means of correcting a humoral shift. Galen rose to fame as a physician caring for the gladiators of Rome. Eventually, he was appointed to the prestigious role of personal physician for emperor, Marcus Aurelius. His skill in treating wounds and controlling bleeding made him a legendary figure. He used styptic agents topically to stop blood loss. Many of Galen's writings have survived to the present day which indicated he was a prolific writer and anatomist. He carried carrying out dissections on pigs as human dissection was illegal and based his theories on anatomy on these dissections. The humoral concept was not fully abandoned until the later part of the 19th century.

Origins of Negative Pressure Wound Therapy (NPWT)

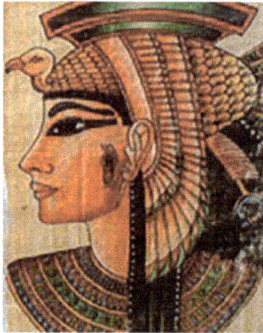

Cleopatra (Image Credit: worldatlas.com)

Penetrating and deeply contaminated wounds were commonly encountered on ancient battlefields, the medical solution for the Roman army was to call in the "wound suckers". These individuals were believed to have hereditary curative powers and used their mouths to suck out debris from the wound beds of injured soldiers. The historian, Suetonius, wrote that a Roman "wound sucker" was deployed to try and revive Cleopatra after she was bitten by the asp. Despite a valiant effort of "lip service" it was ultimately an unsuccessful venture. This mode of treatment would evolve through the ages from the mouth-based technique to using mechanical suction devices for negative pressure wound therapy.

Ancient Skin Grafting

In modern times using skin grafts to heal wounds and burns are quite common. There are autografts (harvested skin from one's own body), allografts (grafts from another human) and xenografts (grafts from another species). It may be a surprise to learn that the earliest skin grafting (autograft) may have occurred around 1500 B.C. in Egypt. Celsus and Galen both made use of skin grafts to address facial injuries in the 1st and 2nd centuries AD. There is some evidence from an ancient Hindu text, that skin grafting was also being used in that region of the world (India) approximately 3,000 years ago. Throughout the Middle Ages there was a lull in graft development potentially due to the disruption of medical learning, but by the 19th century this surgical intervention underwent a revival.

Influence of Islam

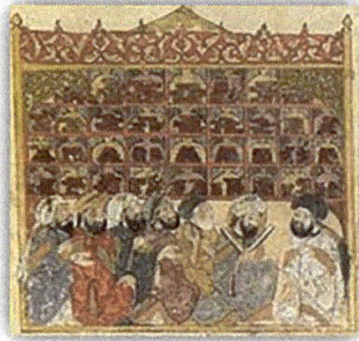

Islamic Golden Age (image credit: en.wikipedia.org)

The Islamic world saw a period of growth and expansion known as the Islamic Golden Age (8th-13th century AD). This epoch showed significant advancement in the areas of mathematics and medicine. Islamic scholars incorporated knowledge from around the world including manuscripts from Greece and China. Islamic tradition encouraged practices of regular handwashing; the practice of quarantining the sickest from the general population, and the establishment of hospitals to care for everyone regardless of socio-economic status. These practices were directly due to religious beliefs but were also advantageous in terms of preventing and treating infectious diseases.

Al Hussain Ibn Abdullah Ibn Sina (Latin name: Avicenna) was the most prominent Muslim physician of this era. He was born in 980 A.D. in present-day Uzbekistan and as child excelled in his academic pursuits. Ibn Sina became a physician and wrote an estimated 450 works on medicine, astronomy, and geometry. He drew upon Galen's humoral concept by adding the elemental components, air, water, fire, and earth. Europeans deemed him the prince of physicians, his *Canon of Medicine* was widely respected across all nations. Avicenna observed diabetic patients with gangrene of the lower extremity and recommended a topical mixture of white turmeric and fenugreek. White turmeric contains both anti-inflammatory and antiseptic qualities and is still prescribed in holistic medicine while fenugreek has had a reputation for various medicinal uses that may cause issues to underlying conditions. Avicenna also used silver as a blood purifier and a cure for bad breath. The Islamic academic prowess continued with the publication of the Kitab Al-Tasrif (Method of Medicine) which was a 30-volume series cataloging diseases along with surgical treatments by Abdul Qasimal-Zahrawi (Albucacis) personal physician to Al-Hakam ruler of Spain.

During the Crusades (11th- 13th centuries AD) the military conflicts between Christians and Muslims for control of the Holy Land provided an opportunity for sharing medical knowledge between these factions. Several of the Christian Military Orders (Saint Lazarus & Saint John) provided medical care to soldiers and civilians alike regardless of religious affiliation. Times of military conflict offered an occasion for medical collaboration.

European Medicine in the Middle Ages

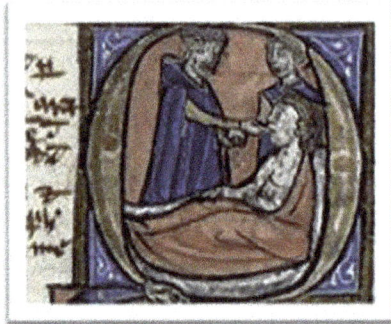

Medieval Medicine (image credit: retrospectjournal.com)

Medicine in medieval Europe (from around 900 CE onward) remained mostly unchanged from that of the Greco-Roman period. The teachings of Claudius Galen persisted as the ultimate medical authority without challenge. Like Islam, Christianity held the belief that caring for the sick was an important religious principle. The Church maintained a stronghold over medicine and surgery during the Middle Ages.

Monks in monasteries diligently copied medical textbooks from ancient Greece and Rome. Monastic hospitals cared for the sick and dying, but the emphasis on hygiene was not as much of a priority as in Islamic medicine. Monks performed procedures such as cautery with a red-hot poker to stop bleeding, bloodletting, and applying leeches to address inflammation of the affected body part. Leeches secrete a natural enzyme which functions as an anticoagulant. Placing a poultice containing wine-soaked cloth would have been a common therapeutic option for skin ulcerations. Many viewed illnesses as a punishment from God and the primary cure was going on a pilgrimage for repentance. Holy shrines and miracle healers were a vital part of any treatment plan through means of securing divine favor. Specific diseases were assigned a particular healing saint, the most prominent examples from this era are Saints Damian (the doctor) and Cosmas (the surgeon). By 1215, the 4th Lateran Council established by Pope Innocent III, decreed it a sacrilege for clergy to withdraw blood from the human body. From that point forward, all surgical procedures were carried out by barbers. Barber surgeons performed limb amputations in the presence of gangrene which was life threatening. The steps of an amputation were as follows; a tourniquet was applied to the diseased limb, an incision was made from skin to bone above the level of necrosis, followed by a serrated bone saw to remove the limb, and lastly the skin was then placed of over the exposed bone, limited closure of the skin, and lastly bandaged into place. The surgical site was cleansed daily, and the amputated limb was displayed as a votive offering in the monastery. The survival rates after amputation were dismal due to the inability to control infection resulting in sepsis.

As the medieval period progressed, some physicians and surgeons dared to question the Galenic tradition. One of these forward thinkers was Henri de Mondeville (1260-1320). This French surgeon was one of the first to write a text regarding the field of surgery. In his treatise, he discussed the treatment of wounds specifically promoting the cleansing of debris from the wound bed and controlling the bleeding with styptic agents. He spoke out against probing the wound to promote pus formation (suppuration) which was believed to be a normal sign of healing. Other physicians felt his views were highly controversial especially for the use of dressings soaked in wine to further prevent pus formation. Despite what some physicians viewed as heretical views; he was appointed as the personal surgeon to King Philip IV (Philip the Fair) of France.

At this time there was a division in the medical field between the academic application and those who practiced medicine on the local level. There was often a gap between the two without sharing knowledge. In part this was because "medicine" was learned through those who could afford the education, while "surgery" where those who handled people and learned through apprenticeship. Henri de Mondeville was a gifted educator who also criticized the class division between medicine (academic) and surgery (trade). This chasm within the medicine profession would continue until the later part of the 18th century.

Another notable medieval French physician, Guy de Chauliac, wrote a popular surgical textbook in 1363 titled, *Cyrurgia Magna* (Great Surgical Work). Chauliac was heavily influenced by Galen but did encourage the removal of foreign bodies from the wounded area along with primary closure of the injury, if possible. The closing of wound edges was deemed a questionable technique in the eyes of conventional medicine during the Medieval age. Chaulic favored tying off or ligating blood vessels to control hemorrhage, this technique would gain popularity in the coming centuries. He was praised for his selfless dedication to treating the sick during the bubonic plague (black death).

Section II: Road to the Renaissance- Challenging Tradition

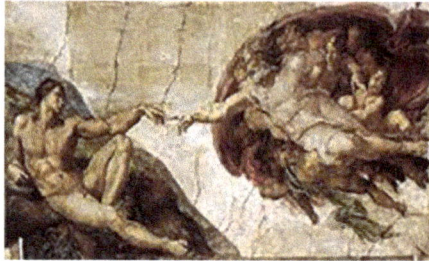

Creation of Man(Image Credit: Britannica.com)

The late Middle Ages into the early Renaissance period (15th -17th centuries) saw growing academic skepticism over the established principles in medicine. One of the most vocal critics of both Galen and Avicenna was Theophrastus Philippus Aureolus Bombastus von Hohenheim (known commonly as Paracelsus), a Swiss physician & alchemist born in 1493. He had a keen interest in botany and chemistry while attending the University of Vienna to become a physician. During his travels around Europe, he disapproved of the common treatment method for ballistic wounds which was to apply boiling oil.

His experience as an alchemist fused into his medical practice where he focused on the health benefits of minerals and metals. He incorporated the use of arsenic, gold, sulfur, silver, lead, copper, and mercury into his care regimen. Paracelsus recommended the application of mercury for the treatment of syphilis and believed that different diseases were associated with specific organs that had corresponding chemical remedies. He was no stranger to controversy, openly expressed his disapproval of both Catholic and Protestant doctrines, and regularly burned Galen's books. Paracelsus is acknowledged as a pioneer of the fields of both pharmacology & toxicology. This widespread questioning of the status quo began the road to further scientific and medical enlightenment.

Advances in Anatomy

Galen's anatomy books were the mainstay for European medical schools in the early 16th century. Human dissections were not specifically outlawed by the Catholic Church during this time, but the work was deemed dirty and a low-class pursuit. Many physicians hired assistants of lower social status to perform these dissections but never questioned Galen's doctrines. This would forever change with the work of Andreas Vesalius, Professor of Surgery, at the University of Padua beginning around 1538. Vesalius dissected cadavers himself against any prevailing social stigma. These bodies were usually freshly executed prisoners from Padua's public gallows. His "hands on" approach along with meticulous notes and artistic anatomical sketches led to the creation of the *De Human Corporis Fabrica Septem Libri* (Seven Books on the Fabric of the Human Body) in 1543. This masterpiece covered the skeleton, musculature, cardio-pulmonary, gastrointestinal, and neurologic organ systems. Vesalius established that the heart was the origin of the inferior vena cava (not the liver, as Galen proposed). He was one of the first to diagnose a dissecting aortic aneurysm. Vesalius' brilliant anatomical manuals were widely read internationally as the invention of the printing press made this possible.

Ballistic Wounds: Lessons from the Battlefield

War despite its cruelty as mentioned before can offer an occasion to improve medical care, and this was the case during the frequent military conflicts in Europe during the Renaissance period. The use of gun powder ushered in the age of ballistic warfare and with it a new challenge for military physicians and surgeons. The standard treatment for ballistic injuries was to cauterize the wounds with boiling oil. It was believed that gunpowder poisoned the wounds, and the only cure was to cauterize the area with scalding oil. French military surgeon, Ambroise Parè, noticed the poor outcomes of patients who were treated with boiling oil including fever and intense pain. To alleviate suffering, he applied a mixture of egg yolks, turpentine, and rose oil to the wounded body part instead of the old standby (hot oil). Parè was pleasantly surprised at the improved condition and survival rate following his new topical regimen. He published his ***Treatise on Gunshot Wounds*** in 1545, which was truly remarkable.

He embraced the principles that a surgeon should be skillful, educated, merciful, kindly to the sick, and honorable while rendering care for patients regardless of their ability to pay. This notion was put forth by his predecessor, Guy de Chauliac (c. 1300-1368). His modesty is reflected in his famous quote "Je le pansai, Dieu le guérit (I bandaged him, God cured him)".

Parè was born of humble origins and thus went the path of the barber surgeon as medicine was still stratified by class with surgery seen as a trade rather than an academic profession. His skill and gentle manner did not go unnoticed, as he was appointed personal master surgeon to four French kings spanning a 30-year period. He developed a clamp called a *bec de Corbin* (crow's beak), to control bleeding from penetrating neck wounds. Ambroise Parè is considered the father of military surgery for his improvement of battlefield medicine and surgery.

Conquering the Circulatory System

Further development of anatomic and wound healing knowledge led to more comprehensive exploration into the complex circulatory system. It was widely accepted that blood formed anew from digested food and the heart's primary function was to produce heat and the lungs moved the blood. The work of English physician, William Harvey, changed these long-held beliefs, demonstrating the true intricacy of human circulation. He performed experiments on living animals to observe the function of heart with the active pumping of blood. Dr. Harvey also noted circulation of blood through the lungs and heart then pumped throughout the body. He described the movement from arterial to venous systems. He was the personal physician to King James I of England and published his exceptional book on the circulatory system in 1628, titled *Exercitatio Anatomica de Motu Cordis et Sanguinis in Animalibus (*Concerning the motion of the heart and blood). He speculated the presence of capillaries which formed junctions between arteries and veins, this was later confirmed in 1661 by Italian physician, Marcello Malpighi.

At the close of the Renaissance in the 17th century, there was a push to re-examine the philosophy behind applying wound dressings. Italian surgeon, Cesare Magati (1579-1647), documented in his work *De rara medicatione vulnerum* (About the rare dressing of wounds) that allowing the wound to rest yielded a better outcome as compared to frequent dressing changes which interrupted healing. He observed this clinical phenomenon during the treatment of a young girl with a chronic leg ulceration, when daily dressing changes resulted in little healing progress. He then changed her dressing every other day and the ulceration finally resolved. These novel views of science and medicine would continue to evolve into the 18th century.

Section III: 18th Century-Time of Innovation

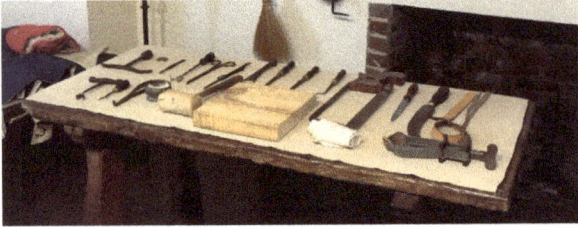

18th Century Surgical Table (Spanish Military Hospital Museum-St. Augustine, Florida)

As the 18th century progressed the class division between medicine and surgery began to dissolve, moving toward a more unified profession. Medical education underwent significant advancement thanks in large part to Dr. Herman Boerhaave (1668-1738). Dr. Boerhaave implemented the concept of bedside teaching into a heavily didactic curriculum. For his clinical approach to teaching, he is credited as the originator of modern medical education.

The field of surgery greatly benefitted from the expanded anatomical knowledge but remained a highly dangerous pursuit. Surgical procedures were performed without any anesthesia and speed was considered the mark of a proficient surgeon. The inability to address infection kept the post-operative mortality rates very high.

It is remarkable that surgeons of the past were able to perform their duties on fully conscious patients knowing the bleak outcome but still hoping to save lives. Limb amputation was the 1st line surgical intervention for any penetrating injury or chronic wound.

Pioneering Hemostasis

An amputation was performed to prevent a fever from setting in and ultimately death from sepsis. To control bleeding during the procedure a tourniquet was applied, most often these were leather straps tied around the extremity. Many patients bled to death due to the tourniquet loosening up as they struggled during the operation. Jean-Louis Petit (1674-1750), a brilliant French surgeon, designed an ingenious device to tackle this hurdle of hemostasis. He developed the "Screw or Petit Tourniquet" that used leather straps with metal clamps that enabled the tourniquet to be locked in place, maintaining vital vessel compression, and allowing the surgeon time to address larger vessels (arteries and veins) through ligation. Though to modern eyes the Screw Tourniquet may seem simplistic in design, it was truly a lifesaving innovation, and is the precursor to the pneumatic tourniquets of today. Jean Louis-Petit wrote several treatises during his lifetime and advocated the use of splints on the leg and foot in an extended position to treat partial Achilles Tendon ruptures, still a contemporary non-operative treatment option. He also felt that breast cancer should be treated aggressively including axilla (underarm) node surgical excision along with mastectomy, that was truly an oncologic concept far head of its time. In terms of wound management, Petit recommended frequent washing with alcohol to promote healing.

Combating Scurvy

From the 16th through 18th century, it is estimated that 2 million sailors died from scurvy, often referred to as the "scourge of the sea". The long sea voyages along with minimal ways to preserve food led to horrible cases of malnutrition. The typical diet of a sailor of that era would be salted meat and biscuits (hardtack). The lack of fresh fruits and vegetables manifested in this hideous illness known as scurvy. Scurvy, a deficiency in vitamin C, leads to poor collagen formation resulting in hemorrhage from friable blood vessels. Common clinical manifestations of scurvy include bleeding gums with tooth loss, non-healing cutaneous (skin) ulcerations of the legs and diffuse joint pain eventually leading to heart failure. A typical 18th century treatment for scurvy was to administer an "elixir of vitriol" (solution of sulfuric acid) along with a round or two of bloodletting. Dr. James Lind, a British naval physician, began an experiment in 1747 to see if he could cure scurvy by use of citrus fruits. He took twelve sailors suffering from scurvy and treated half of them with the standard of care (elixir of vitriol) as the control group, the other half received two oranges and one lemon per day. After one week of treatment, those sailors consuming citrus fruits showed significant signs of recovery.

Dr. Lind published his "Treatise of the Scurvy" in 1753, unfortunately it took the British Navy over 42 years to put it into clinical practice by distributing lemon juice routinely to sailors. For vanquishing the "scourge of the sea", he is generally seen as the father of naval medicine.

Healing & The American Revolution (1775-1783)

The 18th century saw sweeping changes not only in scientific matters but also in the political arena. The American colonies openly rebelling against the British Empire would call into question the established order which had prevailed for centuries. The formation of a new nation had many challenges especially the lack of formal medical education available in the colonial frontier. Colonial physicians for the most part received training solely through the apprentice system which created inconsistency in the standard of care. The most prestigious institutions of medical education were largely based in Europe (Scotland, France, and Italy). Philadelphia was the center of the medical community in the thirteen American colonies with the first hospital being established there in 1751. The Philadelphia College of Medicine founded in 1765 was the first medical school in the thirteen American colonies. Dr. John Jones (1729-1791) was born in New York and pursued his formal medical studies in France. He returned home to practice medicine and served in the French & Indian War (1756-1763). His surgical talents were recognized and praised widely. After the war in 1767, he was instrumental in founding the King's College of Medicine (which would later become Columbia University). When the American Revolution began, Dr. Jones wrote the first American surgical textbook, *Plain Concise Practical Remarks on the Treatment of Wounds and Fractures* in 1777. His work laid out practical techniques for managing acute wounds by bringing the skin edges together and applying adhesive plasters (linen strips with sturgeon bladder adding a gluey quality), these are the forerunner of contemporary steri-strips. He advocated for limb amputation as a last resort for the worst cases of trauma including open fractures.

His surgical textbook was used consistently by military surgeons throughout the War of Independence. Dr. Jones' most famous patients included both Benjamin Franklin and George Washington. For his dedication to medical education and surgical practice, he is regarded as the father of American surgery.

Another notable 18th century American physician was Dr. Benjamin Rush (1745-1813), he received his formal medical degree from the University of Edinburgh in 1766. Dr. Rush became teaching faculty at the Philadelphia College of Medicine and was a signer of the

Declaration of Independence. He was a strong advocate for providing care to the poor and the mentally ill. His strong convictions and personality often put him at odds with colleagues including an extremely adversarial relationship with George Washington.

18th Century Wound Care & Negative Pressure Wound Therapy (NPWT)

Towards the close of the 18th century famous Scottish surgeon, Benjamin Bell (1749-1806) published a textbook devoted to wound healing in 1777 titled, *A treatise on the theory and management of ulcers: with a dissertation on white swellings of the joints*. Dr. Bell's work offered treatment options for various cutaneous wounds and even those associated with "white swellings" archaic term associated with tuberculosis that affected the musculoskeletal system. In the chart below, Bell's remedies are based off characteristics of conditions within the wound itself, including the presence of erythema (redness), moisture/drainage, dryness, and the type of tissue present on clinical examination:

Dr. Benjamin Bell's *Treatise on the Management Ulcers, 1777*

Wound Type	Treatment
Painful wound with redness (ery-thema)	Goulard's cerate "soothing application" of oil, whale wax, and lead
Hyper-granular (excessive vascular tissue formation)	Lunar Caustic (silver nitrate)
Macerated (dampness in wound bed)	Escharotics- drying agent such as Bloodroot
Sinus Tracts (tunneling)	Cords of cottons
Callus formation	Emollients-softening agents
White Swelling (septic arthritis associated with tuberculosis)	Mercury topically with blood-letting

It is interesting to note that silver nitrate is still used to treat hyper-granular tissue and moisture balance remains a tenet of wound healing. The use of lead and mercury were quite common in the 18th century to balance humors as they caused excessive sweating and salivation.

During the 18th century, the "lip service" approach to wound treatment from the Roman era began to lose favor. A French Surgeon, Dominique Anel, found the act of "wound sucking" to be particularly grotesque.

His disdain for this practice inspired him to invent the suction syringe with a triangular tip and a large cannula. The tool was effective in draining abscesses and hematomas. The suction syringe was a more pleasant and safer alternative to the mouth-to-wound method to achieve negative pressure therapy.

From Inoculation/Variolation to Vaccination

Smallpox, the deadly variola virus, tormented mankind for centuries, claiming lives across all nations and socio-economic groups. This disease was often referred to as the "speckled monster" as it left its survivors deeply scarred and disfigured. The fatality rate of smallpox during the 18th century was as high as 60% and amongst infants it was even higher. It was well understood that those who contracted smallpox but survived became immune to the disease. The practice of inoculation was the best means to combat this "speckled monster", and was broadly used in Africa, India, and China for centuries before being introduced to Europe by the early 1700's. Inoculation is derived from the Latin word *inoculare*, meaning "to graft". This procedure consisted of harvesting a small amount of fluid from a smallpox-stricken individual's pus filled sore and then invasively introduced into a healthy person's skin. There was much skepticism in Europe about this risky practice, but ultimately this endeavor paid off. Inoculation also termed variolation (specific to the smallpox virus) significantly reduced the fatality rate as compared to those who contracted the infection naturally.

British physician and scientist, Edward Jenner (1749-1823), had a keen interest in biology and the seemly protective nature of cowpox against the menace of smallpox. He began clinical experimentation on dairymaids, harvesting fluid from cowpox lesions and inoculating them into healthy patients. The patients developed a mild fever and other minor symptoms but recovered completely. Afterwards these patients showed no signs of illness when inoculated later with smallpox. In 1798, Dr. Jenner published, *An Inquiry into the Causes and Effects of the Variolae Vaccinae*, he named this new treatment vaccination from the Latin words for cow *"Vacca"* and *cowpox vaccinae.* This extraordinary discovery of the cowpox vaccine finally gave humanity a solid defense against the formidable enemy of smallpox. In the next century, the power of vaccination is more fully explored along with the acceptance of germ theory.

The 18th century saw innovations in medicine including a better method of controlling bleeding and finally overcoming dreaded diseases such as scurvy and smallpox. Some topical wound healing treatments from this epoch have stood the test of time while other have faded out of favor. The spirit of change in the form of revolution also permeated the fabric of the 18th century mindset.

Section IV: 19th Century- The Advent of Antiseptics & Anesthesia

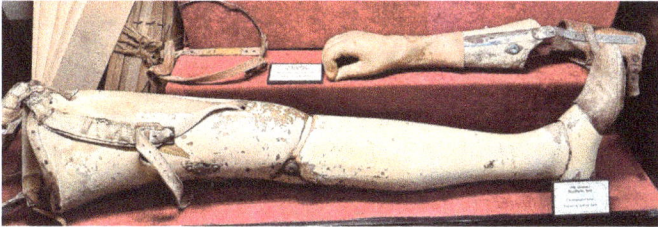

Late 18th through Early 19th Century Prosthetic Devices (Spanish Military Hospital Museum-St. Augustine, FL)

During 19th century a major shift took place with the discovery of anesthesia and the acceptance of germ theory which finally ended the long reign of Galenic influence on clinical medicine. Surgical success was no longer based off mere speed due to the availably of anesthesia, so operative skill received far more attention. The use of antiseptics provided the first steps in combating infection, saving many more lives and limbs than in previous centuries.

19th Century Debridement & Efficient Care Coordination

Once again, the battlefield would be the birthplace of medical progress during the early part of the

19th century. The Napoleonic Wars (1803-1815) were a major global conflict and the horrific sight of wounded soldiers left to die unattended on the battlefield was indeed a tragedy. Dominique Jean Larrey, French surgeon, saw firsthand the catastrophic effect of delayed care to the seriously injured. He astutely recommended immediate surgical intervention for traumatic wounds including debridement (removal of devitalized tissue) and amputation (for severe injuries) which resulted in a better survival rate. He and fellow French surgeon, Pierre Joseph Desault (1744-1795), are credited for coining the term "debridement" referring to the unbridling of flesh. Dominique Larrey also noted the healing advantages of using maggots to assist in removing dead matter from wounds during a military campaign in Egypt.

To prevent soldiers from being left behind languishing, he established an organized system of evacuation for the wounded. This initiative would be named "les ambulances volantes" or "flying ambulances", where skilled medics were dispatched with equipment to render emergent care and evacuate the injured in an efficient manner utilizing horse drawn carts. Napoleon embraced this new method of caring for causalities and it became a standard procedure in the French army.

The "flying ambulance" model would be implemented later during the American Civil War (1861-1865). The Union and Confederate armies faced similar obstacles regarding the evacuation of wounded soldiers during the 1st Battle of Bull Run in 1861, where 5,000 soldiers lay stranded for up to one week after the fighting had ceased. Major General George McClellan appointed Dr. Jonathan Letterman, as Medical Director of the Army of the Potomac in the summer of 1862, chosen for his organizational skills and tasked with improving overall care coordination in the Union army. Dr. Letterman's plan had each regiment supported by 3 dedicated ambulances (horse drawn carts) each with 2 privates and a driver. His plan required a surgeon, and an assistant to assess the patients and decided the appropriate level of care required, which is known today as "triage" a French term meaning "to sort". Those with minor injuries were treated at "first aid" stations and returned to fighting while the more critically wounded were transported to field hospitals beyond cannon range. This method of triage was the basis for Mobile Army Surgical Hospitals (MASH) units implemented in the 20th century and its tenets are still observed in modern emergency departments and trauma centers.

Introduction of Anesthesia

The field of surgery and humanity in general breathed a sigh of relief during the 1840's when inhalable anesthetic agents were finally discovered. Ether is colorless, flammable, and pleasant-smelling liquid first used as anesthetic agent by Boston dentist, Dr. William Thomas Green Morton in 1846. After viewing Dr. Morton's surgical demonstration with ether, Dr. Oliver

Wendell Holmes suggested the use of the term "anesthesia" for this process rendering a patient unconscious to spare them pain, based off the Greek word "anaisthesis" meaning loss of sensation.

Chloroform is a colorless, sweet smelling and nonflammable liquid first used by Scottish obstetrician, Dr. James Young Simpson, during a difficult delivery due to severely contracted pelvis in 1847. Chloroform takes effect quicker than ether but also a greater risk for fatal overdoses. Despite these pitfalls, the age of anesthesia ended the suffering and terror of the surgical theatre.

Birth of the Antiseptic Age

Louis Pasteur's groundbreaking discovery of germ theory (1857) centering around the world of microbes, was the catalyst to finally abandon Claudius Galen's humoral theory of disease. Pasteur's work began the field of microbiology and laid the foundation for the future study of virology with the term "virus" derived from Latin word meaning "poison". He is also credited with developing the earliest vaccines for rabies and anthrax. Pasteur's new findings would not immediately crossover into the clinical realm, indeed acceptance of innovation can be a frustratingly sluggish process.

Dr. Ignaz Semmelweis, a Hungarian physician, struggled with the high mortality rate due to childbed fever on his maternity ward. He noted that midwives had better survival rates than those delivered by physicians. Dr. Semmelweis speculated that the handling of corpses between deliveries played a part in the dire outcomes. He instituted a policy of hand washing with a solution of chloride of lime (calcium hypochlorite) in between each delivery and noted a huge reduction in fever deaths. In 1861, he published a book, *"The Etiology, Concept, and Prophylaxis of Childbed Fever"*, that was ridiculed and rejected by the medical community. Dr. Semmelweis never recovered from this backlash and died in an insane asylum, today he is recognized as the savior of mothers.

Dr. Joseph Lister, a British surgeon, took the scientific theory of Louis Pasteur and implemented it into clinical medicine by theorizing that non-healing wounds after debridement occurred because of the environment within the wound itself, not from miasmas "foul air" which was the standard explanation of that time. Dr. Lister in 1867 inspired by germ theory began using carbolic acid (phenol) as a disinfectant on all surgical wounds and found a huge improvement in healing outcomes, thus officially beginning the age of antiseptic use. He is viewed as the father of modern surgery with the antiseptic mouthwash, Listerine, named in his honor. Russian surgeon, Carl von Reyher (1846-1890), implemented the use antiseptics after cleaning out of wounds resulted in positive outcomes during the Russo-Turkish Wars. Pasteur and Lister's contributions helped humanity finally have a grasp on handling the fatal grip of infection but there was still much ground to cover.

The next phase would be championed by the Prussian physician, Dr. Robert Koch. Building upon the work of his predecessors, Dr. Koch identified the following pathogens, *Staphylococcus* (common causative bacteria in wound infections) and *Vibrio cholera* (cholera) bacterium. In 1882, he achieved a medical milestone by identifying *tubercle bacillus* the causative agent of Tuberculosis. Tuberculosis was a lethal malady that besieged mankind for centuries, and in recognition of this discovery he won the Nobel Prize in 1905.

Development of the Unna Boot
(Soothing Compression)

Using cloth bandages to provide compression in wound healing goes back to ancient times, but towards the end of the 19th century a new innovative paste dressing was created. Paul Gerson Unna, German dermatologist, developed a special dressing to treat venous leg ulcerations with associated dermatitis (skin inflammation) in 1885. This gauze bandage contained zinc oxide in a gelatinous paste that stiffened over time. The Unna boot provided continuous compression while alleviating itching of the skin. Today, Unna boots a staple in the treatment of venous leg wounds in the presence of venous stasis dermatitis.

19ᵗʰ Century Skin Grafting & NPWT

The availability of anesthesia provided the opportunity for further surgical experimentation with skin grafting procedures to accelerate wound healing. In 1869, Dr. Jaques-Louis Reverdin, Swiss surgeon, successful achieved free grafting by harvesting skin from the arm of a patient and implanting it in their wound bed. A year later, a pediatric burn patient received grafts harvested from her abdomen to cover a large skin defect on her thigh by Dr. Georg David Pollock, a British surgeon.

Split-thickness skin grafts contain both epidermis (top layer of skin) and dermis (layer with blood vessels) and was introduced by Dr. Louis Leopold Ollier, French surgeon, in 1872. This new grafting technique demonstrated faster healing and less scar formation. In 1886, Dr. Carl Thiersch introduced his split-thickness grafting technique by harvesting razor thin pieces of epidermis along with bits of dermis attached. To honor both surgeons and their similar inventive skin grafting procedures, the method was officially named the "Ollier-Thiersch graft".

Negative pressure wound therapy (NPWT) took the form of cupping throughout the 19ᵗʰ century. Cupping is a technique of putting heated cups on the skin to create suction. Dr. Francis Fox, British physician, invented the "Glass Leech" that was a suction apparatus with a wide neck cup and adhered to the skin much like a leech in 1821. Dr. Gustav Bier implemented a cupping system that included tubing and a bulb around 1890. This allowed for wound secretions to be extracted in an efficient and contained manner.

Early Hyperbaric Oxygen Therapy (HBOT)

Experimentation with the restorative value of pressurized oxygen chambers occurred as early as 1662 when British physician Nathaniel Henshaw utilized one called a *domicilium* to treat digestive and respiratory illnesses. During the 19th century, a resurgence of interest in hyperbaric medicine took place as Dr. Junod, a French physician, constructed a chamber to treat pulmonary disorders subsequently noting an improvement in patients' blood circulation because of this modality.

The first hyperbaric chamber in the United States was constructed in 1861 by neurologist, James Leonard Corning. He used hyperbaric therapy to help workers suffering from decompression sickness while constructing the Hudson tunnel. Greater understanding of pressurized oxygen and its effect on the human body was established by French physiologist, Paul Bert in 1878. He is recognized as the father of hyperbaric physiology for his research in the treatment of Caisson's disease (nitrogen bubbles in the blood). Hyperbaric medicine and its therapeutic offerings for wound healing would evolve in the next century.

Progression in Understanding Diabetes

During the early part of the 19th century, it was commonly believed that glucose was transported through the lymphatic system into the blood where it was burned off. The talented French physiologist, Claude Bernard, was skeptical of the prevailing theory and began animal experimentation in the search for scientific clarity. In 1848, his published work "About the Origin of Sugar", established the glycogenic (glucose storage) action of the liver. Not long after German pathologist and physiologist, Paul Langerhans (1847-1888), began studying cross sections of pancreatic tissue under microscopy around 1869, discovering cells that would later be recognized as responsible for insulin production (pivotal for regulating blood glucose). The "Islets of Langerhans" were named in his honor after his early death at the age of 40 from tuberculosis.

Another defining moment in the understanding of diabetes occurred at the close of the 19th century with the research of German physicians/physiologists, Drs. Oskar Minkowski, and Joseph Von Mering through experimentation on dogs. They validated that the pancreas was responsible for the maintenance of glucose homeostasis (equilibrium) and crucial to the pathogenesis of diabetes. There was still no effective treatment for diabetes at this point, the only option was to limit dietary intake of carbohydrates as means to control blood glucose levels. Many diabetic patients had shortened life spans due to the lack of effective therapeutic treatment.

Significant headway was made in the awareness of infectious diseases along with the advent of anesthesia providing an environment for surgical advancement in the 19th century. One such milestone was the first heart operation conducted in 1896. Continued research in cellular physiology and pathology blossomed with Dr. Rudolph Virchow (1821-1912) discovering the role of white blood cells in the inflammatory process and the true reason for suppuration (pus formation). Modern medicine's roots are firmly planted in the progress of the 19th century.

Section V: 20th Century to the Present

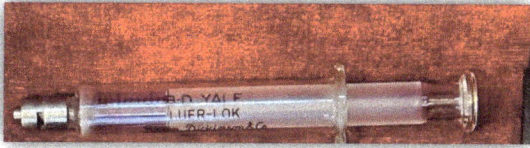

1960's Insulin Syringe (Spanish Military Hospital Museum-St. Augustine, Florida)

At the dawn of the 20th century, the widespread use of antiseptics gave way to aseptic surgical technique where cleanliness standards emphasized the sterilization of instruments and the wearing of masks, gloves, and gowns. In 1901, a significant advancement in the treatment of hemorrhage took place with the recognition of blood groups and compatibility by Dr. Karl Landsteiner, making transfusions much safer. The addition of sodium citrate prevented clot formation and prolonged the overall shelf life of the blood bank. Medical education in the United States transitioned from the unregulated profit driven model to standardized scientific knowledge-based institutions with set admissions criteria as outlined in the Flexner Report 1910.

Anesthesia would expand from the inhalable agents of the 19th century to injectable and intravenous anesthetics as the century advanced. The introduction of clinical X-ray enhanced the diagnosis and treatment of bone diseases, foreign bodies, and fractures. Radiography would aid in the shift from limb amputation to limb preservation during World War I. The modern concepts of addressing moisture balance, infection control, tissue management, and adequate circulation took shape as the 20th century continued.

Progress from World War I (1914-1918)

The battlefield wounds of the First World War were regularly treated with antiseptics, but the heavily manured soil in the trenches of Western Europe served as a breeding ground for deadly gas forming bacteria that was not as susceptible to carbolic acid (phenol). French surgeon, Alexis Carrel, and English chemist, Henry Dakin, combatted this new virulent threat by developing a solution of sodium hypochlorite to irrigate wounds after surgical debridement which killed most bacteria without damaging healthy tissue. The ability to control this aggressive infectious process quite literally saved many lives from the perils of trench warfare. The Carrel-Dakin Method, due to its success, was widely adopted throughout Europe. Dakin's Solution is still used as an antiseptic agent today in wound care.

Battlefield evacuation of the wounded evolved greatly with the use of trains and vehicles but did resemble earlier models seen in the Napoleonic era of the "Flying Ambulances". The efficient access to surgical intervention led to the formation of specialized field hospitals including those dedicated specifically to orthopaedic surgery, plastic surgery, and neurosurgery. The legacy of care designation persists today with specialized units within general hospitals. Treating traumatic wounds previously resulted in amputation, but with improved antiseptics, anesthesia, and radiography limb salvage was a feasible option.

Chemical warfare during World War I was devastating due to mustard gas, a powerful blistering agent, that caused burns to the skin, blindness, and severe irritation of the respiratory system. Research following World War I studied the long-term effects of mustard gas exposure and noted that it suppressed the development of white blood cells. This phenomenon was applied to rapidly dividing cells in patients with lymphoma which began the age of chemotherapy in the 1930s. War again proved to be the catalyst for medical innovation.

Age of Antibiotics

The antibiotic era truly began in the late 19th century into the early 20th century with the work of Dr. Paul Ehrlich (1854-1915) evaluating the antibacterial effects of dyes. He developed stains for histological examination including the basis of the Gram's stain and Ziehl-Neelson stain for tuberculosis.

Dr. Alexander Fleming served in the British army during World War 1 and was dismayed by the infection related deaths of soldiers despite being treated with antiseptics. His research focused on tackling the menace of anaerobic bacterial infections associated with deep wounds. In 1928, Dr. Fleming began experimenting with the staphylococcal bacteria that became contaminated with mold spores. He noticed that the presence of mold caused the death of the bacterial colonies. This species of mold was identified as a member of the *Penicillium* genus, and thus penicillin was born. Penicillin was able to be mass produced by the time of World War II (1939-1945). Around 1935, sulfonamides (sulfa drugs) were discovered by Gerhard Domagk and were very effective again many bacterial diseases. The introduction of antibiotics finally gave humanity a reliable means of treating infections caused by specific pathogens.

Diabetes Treatment: Invention of Insulin

The treatment of diabetes in the beginning of the 20th century still revolved around strict monitoring of dietary intake to control blood glucose. An American physician, Dr. Elliot Joslin, wrote a textbook in 1916, *The Treatment of Diabetes Mellitus* where he emphasized blood sugar control through scientific menu plans including a low carbohydrate diet. Dr. Joslin also felt it was important to empower patients through education to participate in their own care and implemented a system of "wandering diabetes nurses" to help patients in their own homes (the basis of current home healthcare). For his dedication to the treatment of diabetes, the Joslin Diabetes Foundation was created in 1968.

Dr. Frederick Banting, Canadian physician, was inspired after reading an autopsy report by Dr. Moses Barron, regarding a patient with a pancreatic duct obstruction where the islet cells were preserved, this led him to ponder can islet cell secretion be isolated?

By 1921 Banting began working with Professor John MacLeod and Dr. Charles Best to extract the secretions from the islet cells which were later named insulin, the Latin word for "island". This groundbreaking discovery was eventually purified for human use and Banting's team won the Nobel Prize 1923. The introduction of insulin drastically improved the life expectancy of diabetic patients.

During the 1950's, oral antidiabetic drugs (sulphonylureas) were designed to assist in blood glucose control and in 1966 the first pancreatic transplantation was performed on a severely ill Type-1 diabetic patient. By 1979, the 1st needle free insulin system had been developed to provide pain-free administration and now inhaled insulin sprays are available. Diabetes remains a formidable opponent to modern healthcare but is a treatable disease thanks to the discovery of insulin.

20th century Skin Grafting/Dermal Substitutes

Split-thickness skin grafting benefitted from the development of new instrumentation to assist in the harvesting procedure, the manual dermatome (instrument to cut thin slices of skin), was introduced by Dr. Earl C. Padgett in 1941. The dermatome was able to surgically excise a graft of "three-quarter" thickness which led to improved incorporation of tissue and overall wound healing. This technique was much more precise than the previous free hand method. Dr. James C. Tanner introduced the "mesh dermatome" which cuts the graft into a mesh allowing for greater expansion which covers more surface area of the wound by 1964. The mesh graft method is well established and still in use for wound healing. Autologous (from same individual) split-thickness grafting is still a gold standard for the loss of skin caused by burns. Full thickness grafting (consists of epidermis and dermis) is utilized for reconstructive surgery in modern burn units.

Allogeneic grafts (taken from a different person but of the same species) are typically harvested from cadavers and either cryogenically or glycerol preserved, this technique came into use during the mid-20th century.

Xenografts (tissue from another species) especially porcine (pig) grafts have been frequently used since the 1960s with great success. There are many xenografts on the market including bovine (cow) and fish which are employed for the care of wounds.

Dermal substitutes have gained popularity of the past 40 years, these are a group of biologic, synthetic or biosynthetic materials that provide coverage for open wounds. The first dermal substitute made an appearance in the 1980's, as a dermal layer of bovine collagen and silicone epidermal layer that was easy to apply surgically and yielded positive results. There are many existing dermal substitutes which provide bioengineered scaffolding and growth factors to accelerate wound closure.

Contending with Peripheral Arterial Disease

Impaired circulation remains a prominent cause of wound development and limb amputation as peripheral arterial disease (PAD) is commonplace in diabetic patients. A method of clinically detecting PAD through noninvasive testing was introduced in the 1950s with the ankle-brachial index (ABI), this is a ratio of systolic blood pressure measurement of the ankle as compared to the systolic measurement in the arm (brachial artery).

Vascular surgery began to tackle the problem of PAD during the 20th century with Dr. Jean Kunlin performing a successful femoral-popliteal arterial bypass surgery using the saphenous vein (in reverse manner) on a patient suffering from a necrotic foot wound in 1948. The bypass procedure entails resecting the damaged segment of artery and replacing it with a vein to improve circulation A synthetic Teflon vascular graft was designed in 1976 for use in bypass surgeries.

A less invasive surgical method of treating arterial compromise was implemented in 1974, by using a balloon tipped catheter to re-open a stenosed (blocked) femoral artery. Balloon angioplasty is widely used treatment for arterial disease. Addressing PAD continues to be a priority in wound healing and limb salvage.

Managing Moisture: Advances in Wound Dressing

At the beginning of the 20th century, the use of antiseptics helped to address wound infections, but managing moisture in the wound bed is a pivotal part of the healing cascade. During the latter part of the 20th century, primary wound dressings made from polyurethane, or a combination of gelatin, pectin, and cellulose started the moist wound care revolution. Moisture balance, pain relief, and improved healing were clinically apparent with the introduction of these dressings. Alginate dressing, derived from algae, are highly absorptive and non-adherent when used to treat heavily draining wounds. Today, these products remain the foundation of wound care product selection in the pursuit of healing.

Hyperbaric Oxygen Therapy (HBOT) in Wound Healing

HBOT was being utilized during the early part of the 20th century for the treatment of divers suffering from Caisson's disease. During WWI, German scientists Bernhard and Heinrech Drager treated divers with decompression sickness effectively with pressurized oxygen. Dr. Orval Cunningham used this modality to treat patients with cardiovascular disease during the 1920s. By the 1960's hyperbaric chambers merged into mainstream medicine and were used to treat pediatric patients with cardiac disease. The growing interest and research in hyperbaric therapy led to the formation of the Undersea and Hyperbaric Medical Society (UHMS) in 1967 which continues to govern the safe practice of hyperbaric medicine.

HBOT currently is approved for 14 indications including diabetic foot wounds with underlying refractory (resistant) osteomyelitis (bone infection) along with necrotizing skin infections and clostridial myonecrosis (gas gangrene). HBOT improves the oxygen delivery to the tissues, enhances the delivery of antibiotic therapy, and promotes angiogenesis (formation of blood vessels) while decreasing inflammation. Oxygen is a critical component at all stages of wound healing (hemostasis, inflammation, proliferation, and tissue remodeling). HBOT is an extremely valuable weapon in the fight for limb preservation.

Modern NPWT

Progress in negative pressure wound therapy during the 20th century would again be driven by military conflict, specifically the Soviet-Afghanistan War (1979-1989). Dr. Nail Bagaoutdinov, Soviet surgeon, began using a negative pressure unit with a foam dressing placed in the bed of infected wounds with a surrounding sealant and suction applied in 1985. The commonly recognized form of NPWT units started in the 1990's with the use of polyurethane foam, sealant, and tubing attached to a mechanical vacuum as pioneered by the team from Wake Forest University School of Medicine.

The therapeutic benefits of NPWT are well recognized including reducing edema, increasing blood flow, and stimulating the formation of granulation tissue. NPWT units are used today across the spectrum of wound care. NPWT has come a long way from the "lip service" of the Roman era.

Contemporary Biosurgery (Larval Therapy)

During World War I, maggot therapy was utilized to treat open fractures and abdominal wounds. Military surgeon, Dr. William S. Baer, conducted an experiment after the war where 21 patients who had wounds with underlying osteomyelitis (bone infection) that failed other treatment methods were exposed to maggots. After a two-month period, all the patients had healed. Maggot therapy remained a popular treatment option for chronic wounds until the 1940's when penicillin and sulfa drugs were in widespread use. A resurgence of interest in larval therapy happened in the United States during the 1990's when Drs. Ronald Sherman and Edward Pechter established a fly culturing facility in California to produce sterile larvae.

In their clinical trials, it was chronicled that maggot therapy was the most efficient form of debridement as compared to all other non-surgical therapies. It is now understood that the mechanism of action regarding larval therapy include the production of natural antimicrobial-like agents, creation of factors that enhance tissue healing by dissolving dead tissue, and the secretion of ammonia which inhibits bacterial growth. Maggot therapy could be the key in battling multidrug resistant infections in the future.

Autolytic & Enzymatic Debridement

The development of occlusive wound dressings that facilitate the body's natural defenses to breakdown damaged tissue is the basis of autolytic debridement. This technique removes nonviable tissue in a less invasive fashion and is used today when surgical debridement is not feasible.

The application of plant enzymes to chemically break down dead flesh in wounds took shape in the 1940's using juice from the papaya. Another group of debriding enzymes with bacterial origins particularly *Clostridium histolyticum* were uncovered in 1951. Clostridial collagenase ointment is presently the only enzymatic debriding agent available in the United States. Collagenase is a very effective means of removing slough from various types of wounds including diabetic foot ulcerations, venous leg ulcerations, pressure injuries, and burns.

The 20th century to the present is indeed an age of technology with bioengineered skin substitutes and composite wound dressing that maintain optimal healing conditions readily available. The use of HBOT and various forms of NPWT have expanded the capacity for healing complex wounds and injuries. Early detection of PAD is now achieved via angiography (medical imaging of blood vessels using a contrast agent). Debridement can be carried out sharply (with a scalpel), using maggot therapy, enzymatically, mechanically, via ultrasound and/or by pressurized saline jet. There are a multitude of therapeutic modalities that physicians and health-care providers can access in the quest for limb salvage.

Conclusion

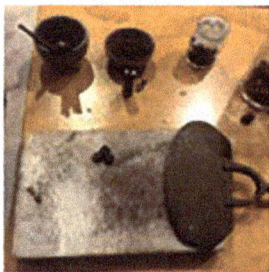

Apothecary Table (Spanish Military Hospital Museum-St. Augustine, Florida)

Looking back at the evolution of wound healing from ancient times to the modern period highlights the ingenuity and perseverance of mankind. In each era, headway was made through clinical observation and scientific exploration despite various obstacles.

The dedication and adaptability of the medical profession is still relevant today as new challenges have arisen including multiple drug resistant organisms (bacteria) and a global pandemic, COVID-19. The emphasis on hand washing and antiseptic use took center stage again during COVID, so a bit of history resurfaced into this 21st century public health crisis.

All contemporary healthcare providers carry on a proud tradition of facing adversity to heal our fellow man. Drawing on the past can give us the fortitude to pursue further medical achievement.

About the Author

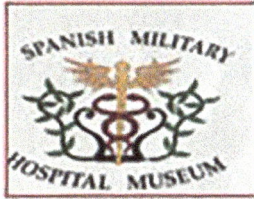

Dr. Christine Miller has a PhD in Christian Crusader Medical History along with specializing in lower extremity wound healing & limb salvage at the University of Florida, College of Medicine-Jacksonville. She has served as the Past Chair of the American College of Clinical Wound Specialists and is currently on the Board of Directors for the Council for America's Military Past (CAMP). Christine is the Chair of the Native American Committee for the Maria Jefferson Chapter of the National Society of the Daughters of the American Revolution (NSDAR). She is a volunteer medical historian for the Spanish Military Hospital Museum in St. Augustine. The love of history and preserving the past is a family affair, her son, Vincent is already a historian training!

Dr. Christine Miller

References

Section I: The Ancient Roots of Healing to the Middle Ages

Alexander, J. W. (2009). History of the medical use of silver. *Surgical Infections*, *10*(3), 289–292. https://doi.org/10.1089/sur.2008.9941

Amr, S. S., & Tbakhi, A. (2007). Ibn Sina (Avicenna) : The Prince of Physicians. *Annals of Saudi Medicine*, *27*(2), 134–135. https://doi.org/10.4103/0256-4947.51520

Bakhtiar, L. (1999). *Avicenna On the Four Humors*. Great Books of the Islamic World, Inc.

Barr, J., Schalick, W. O., & Shortell, C. K. (2020). Surgeons in the time of plague: Guy de Chauliac in four-teenth-century France. *Journal of Vascular Surgery Cases, Innovations and Techniques*, *6*(4), 657–658. https://doi.org/10.1016/j.jvscit.2020.07.006

Forrest, R. D. (1982). Early history of wound treatment. *Journal of the Royal Society of Medicine*, *75*(3), 198–205. https://doi.org/10.1177/014107688207500310

Grens, K. (2019, October 1). Wine therapy, middle ages. *The Scientist, Exploring Life, Inspiring Innovation*, 1–3.

Clarke, C. C. (1931). Henri De Mondeville. *Yale Journal of*

Biology and Medicine, *3*, 459–477.

Hernigou, P., Hernigou, J., & Scarlat, M. (2021). The dark age of medieval surgery in France in the first part of middle age (500–1000): Royal Touch, wound suckers, bizarre medieval surgery, Monk Surgeons, Saint Healers, but foundation of the oldest worldwide still-operating hospital. *International Orthopaedics*, *45*(6), 1633–1644. https://doi.org/10.1007/s00264-020-04914-1

Hernigou, P., Hernigou, J., & Scarlat, M. (2021a). Medieval surgery (eleventh–thirteenth century): Barber Surgeons and Warfare Surgeons in France. *International Orthopaedics*, *45*(7), 1891–1898. https://doi.org/10.1007/s00264-021-05043-z

Kohlhauser, M., Luze, H., Nischwitz, S. P., & Kamolz, L. P. (2021). Historical evolution of skin grafting—a journey through time. *Medicina*, *57*(4), 348. https://doi.org/10.3390/medicina57040348

Laios, K., Karamanou, M., Saridaki, Z., & Androutsos, G. (2012). Aretaeus of Cappadocia and the first description of diabetes. *Hormones*, *11*(1), 109–113. https://doi.org/10.1007/bf03401545

Lakhtakia, R. (2013). The History of Diabetes Mellitus. *Sultan Qaboos University Medical Journal*, *13*(3), 368–370.

Metwaly, A. M., Ghoneim, M. M., Eissa, Ibrahim. H., Elsehemy, I. A., Mostafa, A. E., Hegazy, M. M., Afifi, W. M., & Dou, D. (2021). Traditional ancient egyptian medicine: A Review. *Saudi Journal of Biological Sciences*, *28*(10), 5823–5832. https://doi.org/10.1016/j.sjbs.2021.06.044

Miller, C. (2012). The history of negative pressure wound therapy (NPWT): From "Lip service" to the modern vacuum system. *Journal of the American College of Clinical Wound Specialists*, *4*(3), 61–62. https://doi.org/10.1016/j.jccw.2013.11.002

Nicoli Aldini, N., Fini, M., & Giardino, R. (2008). From Hippocrates to tissue engineering: Surgical Strategies in Wound treatment. *World Journal of Surgery*, *32*(9), 2114–2121. https://doi.org/10.1007/s00268-008-9662-1

Singh, O., Khanam, Z., Misra, N., & Srivastava, M. K. (2011). Chamomile (Matricaria Chamomilla L.): An overview. *Pharmacognosy Reviews*, *5*(9), 82–95. https://doi.org/10.4103/0973-7847.79103

Sipos, P., Győry, H., Hagymási, K., Ondrejka, P., & Blázovics, A. (2004). Special wound healing methods used in ancient Egypt and the mythological background. *World Journal of Surgery*, *28*(2), 211–216. https://doi.org/10.1007/s00268-003-7073-x

Tsiompanou, E., & Marketos, S. G. (2013). Hippocrates: Timeless still. *Journal of the Royal Society of Medicine*, *106*(7), 288–292. https://doi.org/10.1177/0141076813492945

Wallner, C., Moormann, E., Lulof, P., Drysch, M., Lehnhardt, M., & Behr, B. (2020). Burn care in the greek and roman antiquity. *Medicina*, *56*(12), 657–666. https://doi.org/10.3390/medicina56120657

Whitaker, I. S., Twine, C., Whitaker, M. J., Welck, M., Brown, C. S., & Shandall, A. (2007). Larval therapy from antiquity to the present day: Mechanisms of action, clinical applications, and future potential. *Postgraduate Medical Journal*, *83*(980), 409–413. https://doi.org/10.1136/pgmj.2006.05

Section II: Road to the Renaissance- Challenging Tradition

Barr, J. (2015). The anatomist Andreas Vesalius at 500 Years Old. *Journal of Vascular Surgery*, *61*(5), 1370–1374. https://doi.org/10.1016/j.jvs.2014.11.080

Dominiczak, M. H. (2013). Andreas Vesalius: His science, teaching, and exceptional books. *Clinical Chemistry*, *59*(11), 1687–1689. https://doi.org/10.1373/clinchem.2012.199968

Fughelli, P., Stella, A., & Sterpetti, A. V. (2019). Marcello Malpighi (1628–1694). *Circulation Research*, *124*(10), 1430–1432. https://doi.org/10.1161/circresaha.119.314936

Michaleas, S. N., Laios, K., Tsoucalas, G., & Androutsos, G.

(2021). Theophrastus Bombastus von Hohenheim (Paracelsus) (1493–1541): The eminent physician and pioneer of toxicology. *Toxicology Reports*, *8*, 411–414. https://doi.org/10.1016/j.toxrep.2021.02.012

Nicoli Aldini, N., Fini, M., & Giardino, R. (2008). From Hippocrates to tissue engineering: Surgical Strategies in Wound treatment. *World Journal of Surgery*, *32*(9), 2114–2121. https://doi.org/10.1007/s00268-008-9662-1

Packard, F. R. (1926). *Life and times of Ambroise Pare (1510-1590)*. Paul B. Hoeber.

Ribatti, D. (2009). William Harvey and the discovery of the circulation of the blood. *Journal of Angiogenesis Research*, *1*(1), 3–4. https://doi.org/10.1186/2040-2384-1-3

Romanovsky, A. A. (1999). Paracelsus on wound treatment. *The Lancet*, *354*(9193), 1910. https://doi.org/10.1016/s0140-6736(05)76881-1

Tanner, A. M., & Weissler, M. C. (2017). Ambroise Pare: The gentle barber-surgeon. *The American College of Surgeons*, 52–55.

Section III: 18th Century-Time of Innovation

Bell, B. (1797). *A treatise on the theory and management of ulcers; with a dissertation on white swelling of the joints*. Thomas & Andrews.

Griesemer, A. D., Widmann, W. D., Forde, K. A., & Hardy, M. A. (2009). John Jones, M.D.: Pioneer, Patriot, and founder of American Surgery. *World Journal of Surgery*, *34*(4), 605–609. https://doi.org/10.1007/s00268-009-0323-9.

Jones, J., Cadwalader, T., & Bell, R. (1776). *Plain concise practical remarks, on the treatment of wounds and fractures; to which is added, an appendix, on camp and military hospitals; principally designed, for the use of young military and naval surgeons, in North America. by John Jones, M.D. professor of surgery, in King's College, New York.*

Harvie, D. I. (2002). *Limeys: The true story of one man's war against ignorance, the establishment, and the deadly scurvy*. Sutton.

Hull, G. (1997). The influence of Herman Boerhaave. *Journal of the Royal Society of Medicine*, *90*(9), 512–514. https://doi.org/10.1177/014107689709000915

Macintyre, I. M. C. (2011). Scientific surgeon of the enlightenment or 'plagiarist in everything': A reappraisal of Benjamin Bell (1749–1806). *The Journal of the Royal College of Physicians of Edinburgh*, *41*(2), 174–181. https://doi.org/10.4997/jrcpe.2011.211.

Markatos, K., Androutsos, G., Karamanou, M., Tzagkarakis, G., Kaseta, M., & Mavrogenis, A. (2018). Jean-Louis Petit (1674–1750): A pioneer anatomist and surgeon and his contribution to orthopaedic surgery and

Trauma Surgery. *International Orthopaedics*, *42*(8), 2003–2007. https://doi.org/10.1007/s00264-018-3978-8.

Miller, C. (2012). The history of negative pressure wound therapy (NPWT): From "Lip service" to the modern vacuum system. *Journal of the American College of Clinical Wound Specialists*, *4*(3), 61–62. https://doi.org/10.1016/j.jccw.2013.11.002

Miller, C. (2016). *A Guide to 18th Century Military Medicine in Colonial America*. CreateSpace Independent Publishing Platform.

Nicoli Aldini, N., Fini, M., & Giardino, R. (2008). From Hippocrates to tissue engineering: Surgical Strategies in Wound treatment. *World Journal of Surgery*, *32*(9), 2114–2121. https://doi.org/10.1007/s00268-008-9662-1.

North, R. L. (2000). Benjamin Rush, MD: Assassin or beloved healer? *Baylor University Medical Center Proceedings*, *13*(1), 45–49. https://doi.org/10.1080/08998280.2000.11927641

Riedel, S. (2005). Edward Jenner and the history of smallpox and vaccination. *Baylor University Medical Center Proceedings*, *18*, 21–25.

Williams, G. (1975). *The age of agony the art of healing 1700-1800*. Constable.

Section IV: 19th Century-The Advent of Antiseptics & Anesthesia

Bause, G. S. (2012). Ether Day's William T. G. Morton. *Anesthesiology*, *117*(1), 1–2. https://doi.org/10.1097/aln.0b013e3182592300

Best, M., & Neuhauser, D. (2004). Ignaz Semmelweis and the birth of infection control. *Quality and Safety in Health Care*, *13*(3), 233–234. https://doi.org/10.1136/qshc.2004.010918

Brewer, L. A. (1986). Baron Dominique Jean Larrey (1766-1842). *The Journal of Thoracic and Cardiovascular Surgery*, *92*(6), 1096–1098. https://doi.org/10.1016/s0022-5223(19)35826-x

Dunn, P. M. (2002). Sir James Young Simpson (1811-1870) and obstetric anaesthesia. *Archives of Disease in Childhood – Fetal and Neonatal Edition*, *86*(3), 207–208. https://doi.org/10.1136/fn.86.3.f207

Jörgens, V., & Grüsser, M. (2013). Happy birthday, Claude Bernard. *Diabetes*, *62*(7), 2181–2182. https://doi.org/10.2337/db13-0700

Karamanou, M., Protogerou, A., Androutsos, G., & Poulako-Rebelakou, E. (2016). Milestones in the history of diabetes mellitus: The main contributors. *World Journal of Diabetes*, *7*(1), 1–17. https://doi.org/10.4239/wjd.v7.i1.1

Kohlhauser, M., Luze, H., Nischwitz, S. P., & Kamolz, L. P.

(2021). Historical evolution of skin grafting—a journey through time. *Medicina*, *57*(4), 348. https://doi.org/10.3390/medicina57040348

Lakhtakia, R. (2014). The legacy of Robert Koch: Surmise, search, substantiate. *Sultan Qaboos University Medical Journal*, *14*(1), 37–41. https://doi.org/10.12816/0003334

Miller, C. (2012). The history of negative pressure wound therapy (NPWT): From "Lip service" to the modern vacuum system. *Journal of the American College of Clinical Wound Specialists*, *4*(3), 61–62. https://doi.org/10.1016/j.jccw.2013.11.002

Nicoli Aldini, N., Fini, M., & Giardino, R. (2008). From Hippocrates to tissue engineering: Surgical Strategies in Wound treatment. *World Journal of Surgery*, *32*(9), 2114–2121. https://doi.org/10.1007/s00268-008-9662-1.

Queen, D., Orsted, H., Sanada, H., & Sussman, G. (2004). A dressing history. *International Wound Journal*, 1(1), 59–77. https://doi.org/10.1111/j.1742-4801.2004.0009.x

Ortega, M. A., Fraile-Martinez, O., García-Montero, C., Callejón-Peláez, E., Sáez, M. A., Álvarez-Mon, M. A., García-Honduvilla, N., Monserrat, J., Álvarez-Mon, M., Bujan, J., & Canals, M. L. (2021). A general overview on the hyperbaric oxygen therapy: Applications, mechanisms and translational opportunities. *Medici-*

ℓ

na, *57*(9), 864–889. https://doi.org/10.3390/medicina57090864

Pitt, D., & Aubin, J.-M. (2012). Joseph Lister: Father of modern surgery. *Canadian Journal of Surgery*, *55*(5), E8–E9. https://doi.org/10.1503/cjs.007112

Place, R. J. (2015). The strategic genius of Jonathan Letterman: The relevancy of the American Civil War to current health care policy makers. *Military Medicine*, *180*(3), 259–262. https://doi.org/10.7205/milmed-d-14-00419

Revie, N. (2021). *Paul Langerhans (1847-1888)*. Insulin to Innovation. Retrieved July 25, 2022, from https://www.insulintoinnovation.ca/100-lives-of-insulin/paul-langerhans

Santa Lucia, G., Snyder, A., Plante, J., Ritter, A., & Elston, D. (2021). Unna boot efficacy in dermatologic diseases. *Journal of the American Academy of Dermatology*, 85(1), 267–269. https://doi.org/10.1016/j.jaad.2020.11.027

Singh, S., & Gambert, S. R. (2014). Hyperbaric Oxygen Therapy: A Brief History and Review of its Benefits and Indications for the Older Adult Patient. *Annals of Long-Term Care*, 1–8.

Smith, K. A. (2012). Louis Pasteur, the father of immunology? *Frontiers in Immunology*, *3*, 1–10. https://doi.org/10.3389/fimmu.2012.00068

Welling, D. R., Burris, D. G., & Rich, N. M. (2010). The influence of Dominique Jean Larrey on the Art and Science of Amputations. *Journal of Vascular Surgery*, *52*(3), 790–793. https://doi.org/10.1016/j.jvs.2010.02.286

Whitaker, I. S., Twine, C., Whitaker, M. J., Welck, M., Brown, C. S., & Shandall, A. (2007). Larval therapy from antiquity to the present day: Mechanisms of action, clinical applications, and future potential. *Postgraduate Medical Journal*, *83*(980), 409–413. https://doi.org/10.1136/pgmj.2006.

White, E. (2019). Carl von Reyher and the origins of debridement. *Wounds UK*, *5*(3), 85–85.

Section V: 20ᵗʰ Century to the Present-Age of Technology

Barton, M., Gruntzig, J., Husmann, M., & Rosch, J. (2014). Balloon angioplasty-the legacy of Andreas Gruntzig, M.D. (1939-1985). *Frontiers in Cardiovascular Medicine*, *1*, 15–40. https://doi.org/10.3389/fcvm.2014.00015

Bickel, M. H. (1988). The development of Sulfonamides (1932—1938) as a focal point in the history of chemotherapy. *Gesnerus*, *45*(1), 67–86. https://doi.org/10.1163/22977953-04501006

Boulton, F. (2015). Blood transfusion and the World Wars. *Medicine, Conflict and Survival*, *31*(1), 57–68. https://doi.org/10.1080/13623699.2015.1023684

Connolly, J. E. (2011). The history of the in situ saphenous vein bypass. *Journal of Vascular Surgery*, *53*(1), 241–244. https://doi.org/10.1016/j.jvs.2010.05.018

Duffy, T. P. (2011, September). *The Flexner report--100 years later*. The Yale journal of biology and medicine. Retrieved December 17, 2022, from https://pubmed. ncbi.nlm.nih.gov/21966046/

Farhud, D. D. (2018). Karl Landsteiner (1868-1943). *Iran Journal of Public Health*, *47*(6), 777–778.

Gould, K. (2016). Antibiotics: From prehistory to the present day. *Journal of Antimicrobial Chemotherapy*, *71*(3), 572–575. https://doi.org/10.1093/jac/dkv484

Gregory, R. T., & Yao, J. S. T. (2013). The first Gore-Tex femoral-popliteal bypass. *Journal of Vascular Surgery*, *58*(1), 266–269. https://doi.org/10.1016/j. jvs.2013.02.246

Heitzmann, W., Fuchs, P. C., & Schiefer, J. L. (2020). Historical perspectives on the development of current standards of care for enzymatic debridement. *Medicina*, *56*(12), 706–714. https://doi.org/10.3390/medicina56120706

Howell, J. D. (2016). Early Clinical Use of the X-Ray. *Transactions of the American Clinical and Climatology Association*, *127*, 341–349.

Johnston, B. R., Ha, A. Y., Brea, B., & Liu, P. Y. (2016). The Mechanism of Hyperbaric Oxygen Therapy in the

Treatment of Chronic Wounds and Diabetic Foot Ulcers. *Rhode Island Medical Journal* , 26–28.

Keyes, Michael, and Rachel Thibodeau. "Dakin Solution (Sodium Hypochlorite)." StatPearls [Internet]., U.S. National Library of Medicine, 5 Apr. 2019, www.ncbi.nlm.nih.gov/books/NBK507916/.

Kohlhauser, M., Luze, H., Nischwitz, S. P., & Kamolz, L. P. (2021). Historical evolution of skin grafting—a journey through time. *Medicina*, *57*(4), 348. https://doi.org/10.3390/medicina57040348

Mandal, D. A. (2019, February 26). *History of chemotherapy*. News. Retrieved December 17, 2022, from https://www.news-medical.net/amp/health/History-of-Chemotherapy.aspx

Miller, C. (2012). The history of negative pressure wound therapy (NPWT): From "Lip service" to the modern vacuum system. *Journal of the American College of Clinical Wound Specialists*, *4*(3), 61–62. https://doi.org/10.1016/j.jccw.2013.11.002

Nicoli Aldini, N., Fini, M., & Giardino, R. (2008). From Hippocrates to tissue engineering: Surgical Strategies in Wound treatment. *World Journal of Surgery*, *32*(9), 2114–2121. https://doi.org/10.1007/s00268-008-9662-1.

Ortega, M. A., Fraile-Martinez, O., García-Montero, C., Callejón-Peláez, E., Sáez, M. A., Álvarez-Mon, M. A., García-Honduvilla, N., Monserrat, J., Álvarez-Mon,

M., Bujan, J., & Canals, M. L. (2021). A general overview on the hyperbaric oxygen therapy: Applications, mechanisms, and translational opportunities. *Medicina, 57*(9), 864–889. https://doi.org/10.3390/medicina57090864

Tan, S. Y., & Tatsumura, Y. (2015). Alexander Fleming (1881–1955): Discoverer of Penicillin. *Singapore Medical Journal, 56*(07), 366–367. https://doi.org/10.11622/smedj.2015105

Tan, S. Y., & Merchant, J. (2017). *Frederick Banting (1891-1941): Discoverer of insulin*. Singapore medical journal. Retrieved July 25, 2022, from https://www.ncbi.nlm.nih.gov/pmc/articles/PMC5331123/

Thomas, A. M. K., & Banerjee, A. K. (2013, May 1). *Military radiology*. OUP Academic. Retrieved December 17, 2022, from https://doi.org/10.1093/med/9780199639977.003.0003

Whitaker, I. S., Twine, C., Whitaker, M. J., Welck, M., Brown, C. S., & Shandall, A. (2007). Larval therapy from antiquity to the present day: Mechanisms of action, clinical applications, and future potential. *Postgraduate Medical Journal, 83*(980), 409–413. https://doi.org/10.1136/pgmj.2006.05

Zimmerman, L. M., & Howell, K. M. (1932). History of Blood Transfusion*. *Annals of Medial History, IV* (5), 415–432.

More publications by Dr. Christine Miller

Common Natural
Herbal   Remedies
of Colonial Florida

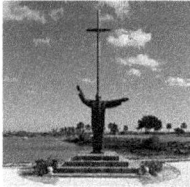

By Dr. Christine Miller

The Royal Spanish
Military Hospital at
Saint Augustine

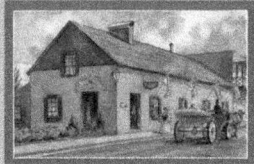

By Dr. Christine Miller

A Guide to 18th Century
MilitaryMedicine in
Colonial America

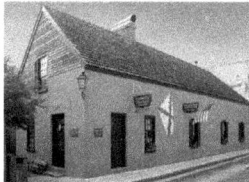

By
Dr. Christine Miller